Fluconazole

The Ultimate Guide to Deal with Vaginal Infections, Yeast Infections, Fungal Meningitis, Throat and Lungs Infections, and Many More Using Fluconazole

Jacob Ryan

Title | Fluconazole
Author | Jacob Ryan
ISBN | 979-12-22751-60-3

© 2024. All rights reserved by the Author
This work is published directly by the Author via the Youcanprint self-publishing platform and the Author holds all rights thereto exclusively. No part of this book may therefore be reproduced without the prior consent of the Author.

Youcanprint
Via Marco Biagi 6, 73100 Lecce
www.youcanprint.it
info@youcanprint.it
Made by human

Copyright ©2024 Jacob Ryan

All rights reserved. No part of this publication may be reproduced, distributed, or transmitted in any form of by any means, including photocopying, recording or other electronic or mechanical methods, without the prior written permission of the publisher, except in the case of brief quotations embodied in critical reviews and certain other noncommercial uses permitted by copyright law.

Legal Disclaimer

The information provided in this book, "Fluconazole - The Ultimate Guide to Deal with Vaginal Infections, Yeast Infections, Fungal Meningitis, Throat and Lungs Infections, and Many More Using Fluconazole" is for general informational and educational purposes only. The author, Jacob Ryan, is not a licensed medical professional, and the content should not be considered a substitute for professional medical advice, diagnosis, or treatment.

Chapter 1: Everything about Fluconazole 7
What is Fluconazole? 7
History of Fluconazole 8
Properties and Characteristics of Fluconazole 8
    Experimental Properties 9
    Predicted Properties 9
    Predicted ADMET Standard 10
What is Fluconazole used for? 11

Chapter 2: Mechanism of Action 13
How does Fluconazole work? 13
Pharmacodynamics 14
Pharmacokinetics 15
Effectiveness of Fluconazole 16

Chapter 3: Warnings, Dosage, and Side Effects 18
Warnings 18
    Allergies 20
    Pediatric 21
    Geriatric 21
    Breastfeeding 22
    Prior to take fluconazole 22
The Proper Dosage 24
Main Side Effects 28
Pharmacist Tips for Fluconazole 32

Chapter 4: Combination with other Medications and Alcohol 34
    Interaction with Alcohol 46

Chapter 5: Pregnancy and Breastfeeding 49
Is it possible and safe to use Fluconazole when pregnant? 49
    Using Fluconazole while Pregnant 49

Using Fluconazole while Breastfeeding 53

Consequences of using Fluconazole when pregnant or breastfeeding 56

Chapter 6: Frequently Asked Questions 58

Chapter 1: Everything about Fluconazole

What is Fluconazole?

In addition to treating vaginal candidiasis, oral thrush, esophageal candidiasis, and other candida infections such UTIs, peritonitis, and inflammation of the stomach lining, fluconazole is also used to treat various types of fungal and yeast infections. This drug will either kill the fungus or yeast, or it will stop its growth and prevent it from spreading.

Patients receiving radiation or chemotherapy and undergoing bone marrow transplants can also use fluconazole to avoid developing candidiasis. A medical requirement of your physician is strictly necessary to buy this drug.

There are different dosing formulations for this product:
- Tablet
- Powder for Suspension

History of Fluconazole

Often sold under the brand name Diflucan, fluconazole is an antifungal medication used to treat both systemic and superficial fungal infections in a wide range of body tissues. Similar to ketoconazole and itraconazole, this medication is an azole antifungal. Advantages of fluconazole over other antifungal medicines include its convenient oral administration. It has been shown to be an effective therapy for vaginal yeast infections with just one dosage.

Properties and Characteristics of Fluconazole

Weight
Average: 306.2708
Monoisotopic: 306.104065446

Chemical Formula
$C_{13}H_{12}F_2N_6O$

State
Solid

Experimental Properties

PROPERTY	VALUE
melting point (°C)	138-140 °C
boiling point (°C)	579.8
water solubility	slightly soluble in water
logP	0.5
pKa	1.76

Predicted Properties

PROPERTY	VALUE
Water Solubility	1.39 mg/mL
logP	0.58
logP	0.56
logS	-2.3
pKa (Strongest Acidic)	12.68
pKa (Strongest Basic)	2.3
Physiological Charge	0
Hydrogen Acceptor Count	5
Hydrogen Donor Count	1
Polar Surface Area	81.65 Å^2
Rotatable Bond Count	5
Refractivity	97.2 m^3·mol^{-1}
Polarizability	26.52 Å^3
Number of Rings	3
Bioavailability	1
Rule of Five	Yes
Ghose Filter	Yes
Veber's Rule	No
MDDR-like Rule	No

Predicted ADMET Standard

PROPERTY	VALUE	PROBABILITY
Human Intestinal Assimilation	+	0.9894
Blood Brain Barrier	+	0.9382
Caco-2 permeable	+	0.8867
P-glycoprotein substrate	Non-substrate	0.6008
P-glycoprotein inhibitor I	Non-inhibitor	0.8782
P-glycoprotein inhibitor II	Non-inhibitor	0.9004
Renal organic cation transporter	Non-inhibitor	0.6461
CYP450 2C9 substrate	Non-substrate	0.7898
CYP450 2D6 substrate	Non-substrate	0.9116
CYP450 3A4 substrate	Non-substrate	0.565
CYP450 1A2 substrate	Non-inhibitor	0.6312
CYP450 2C9 inhibitor	Non-inhibitor	0.5497
CYP450 2D6 inhibitor	Non-inhibitor	0.809
CYP450 2C19 inhibitor	Inhibitor	0.532
CYP450 3A4 inhibitor	Non-inhibitor	0.8196
CYP450 inhibitory crowding	Low CYP	0.524
Ames test	Non AMES toxic	0.548
Carcinogenicity	Non-carcinogens	0.7298
Biodegradation	Not ready biodegradable	1.0

Rat severe toxicity	2.4136 LD50, mol/kg	Not applicable
hERG inhibition (predictor I)	Weak inhibitor	0.8229
hERG inhibition (predictor II)	Non-inhibitor	0.6614

What is Fluconazole used for?

Fluconazole is an antifungal medication for the treatment of yeast infections that manifest in the vaginal cervix, mouth and throat, esophagus, abdomen, lungs, blood, and also other parts of body. The antifungal medication fluconazole is also effective in treating fungal meningitis, which is an infection of the membranes that surround the brain and spine. Individuals who are at a high risk of acquiring fungal infections as a result of chemotherapy or radiation therapy are administered fluconazole prior to undergoing a bone marrow transplant. Fluconazole is a fungicidal medication that belongs to the triazole class. It does this by preventing the growth of the fungus, which is how it fights diseases that are caused by fungus.

Fluconazole is not only used to treat fungal infections, but it is also sometimes prescribed as a preventative measure for people who are at a high risk of developing fungal infections, such as those who have immune systems that are compromised as a result of HIV/AIDS, cancer treatment, or a recent organ transplant. See your doctor for any doubt or concerns about the possible adverse effects of taking this drug.

Chapter 2: Mechanism of Action

How does Fluconazole work?

When it comes to fungi, fluconazole is a potent and specific inhibitor of the lanosterol 14--demethylase that is cytochrome P450 dependent. The usual function of this enzyme is to transform lanosterol into ergosterol, which is required for the formation of the cell wall in fungi. Fluconazole inhibits the activity of lanosterol 14--demethylase by binding to the lone iron atom in the heme group of the enzyme. The nitrogen atom on the azole ring of fluconazole is free. It stops ergosterol production by blocking oxygen activation, which in turn hinders demethylation of lanosterol. Fungal development is stopped once methylated sterols build up in the membrane of the fungus. The accumulation of these sterols disrupts the normal functioning of the plasma membrane of fungal cells.

To develop resistance to fluconazole, the target enzyme (lanosterol 14--demethylase) may undergo changes in expression, activity, or accessibility. Researchers are looking at the possibility that other systems are involved as well.

Pharmacodynamics

Fungal infections can be treated with fluconazole since it has been shown to have fungistatic efficacy against the majority of strains of the following microorganisms:

Yeasts like Candida albicans, Aspergillus niger (Many strains are intermediately susceptible), Cryptococcus neoformans, Candida parapsilosis, and Candida tropicalis.

To treat fungal infections and associated symptoms, steroids are used to decrease fungal cell functions such cell wall formation and growth and cell adhesion.

The antifungal effects of fluconazole have been demonstrated in both healthy and immunocompromised animal models of systemic and intracranial fungal infections generated by Cryptococcus neoformans and systemic infections caused by Candida albicans. It is worth noting that fluconazole-resistant strains of a variety of species have been discovered. This adds more weight to the need for doing susceptibility testing whenever fluconazole is being evaluated as an antifungal treatment option.

Concerns have been raised that fluconazole suppression of hepatic cytochrome enzymes might lead to the disruption and inactivation of human steroids and hormones. The plasma concentrations of testosterone and steroids in both sexes were shown to be unaffected by daily administration of 50 mg of fluconazole to adults (aged 18-35) for up to 28 days. According to one clinical trial cited by the European Medicines Agency label, fluconazole at a dosage range of 200–400 mg had no meaningful effect on steroid standard or on ACTH–response to steroid stimulation in healthy males.

Pharmacokinetics

Whether fluconazole is administered orally or intravenously, its pharmacokinetics are the same. Concentrations reach a maximum around 2 hours after dose, and the oral bio availability is more than 90%. 0.7 L/kg is the apparent volume of distribution, whereas plasma protein binding is just 12%. The medication has a high metabolic stability, with roughly 80% of its elimination occurring as unmodified drug via renal excretion. After 7 days of once-daily dosage, plasma levels had stabilized and increased by around 2.5-fold. Concentrations in the blood plasma are proportionate to the dose, and the elimination half-life is unaffected by either the dose or the passage of time. Fluconazole has a half-life in plasma of around 30 hours. Both healthy old and young persons have comparable pharmacokinetics; however those with renal impairment will need a different dosage.

The CSF, sputum, and saliva are the most permeable to fluconazole, whereas the urine and skin have the highest concentrations.

Effectiveness of Fluconazole

Clinical studies of fluconazole assessed its effectiveness in treating systemic fungal infections in a randomized, controlled setting without any direct comparison. Forty-eight people with confirmed or probable fungal infections were recruited, and their success could be measured. Ninety percent of the fungal infections were caused by Candida albicans. Infections were traced to four different types of yeast: Candida parapsilosis, Candida glabrata, Histoplasma capsulatum, and Aspergillus fumigatus. For an average of 15 days, patients were given a dose of 200-400 mg of fluconazole daily. More than half (53%) of those treated with fluconazole saw improvement. There was a clinical and mycological response in 62% and 65% of patients, respectively, having Candida albicans infections that were either proved or probable. Elevated liver enzymes were suspected to be related to fluconazole treatment in 11 patients, but no adjustments were required in these cases.

After testing, fluconazole was determined to be safe and effective against systemic Candida albicans infections.

Chapter 3: Warnings, Dosage, and Side Effects

Warnings

To ensure this medication is working properly, it is crucial that your doctor monitor your or your child's development at frequent appointments. Tests of the blood and urine may be necessary to detect any adverse reactions.

Because of the potential for dangerous interactions, you or your child should not use erythromycin (Ery-Tab), pimozide (Orap), or quinidine (Cardioquin) at the same time as this medication.

Long-term or excessive use of this medication, especially in the first trimester of pregnancy, might be harmful to the developing fetus. It is recommended that you use a reliable method of birth control during your treatment with this medication and for at least a week after you stop using it. If in the meanwhile you discover a pregnancy, call immediately your doctor.

There have been highly isolated reports of this medicine causing deadly liver damage in some patients. Get in touch with your medical practitioner as quick as possible if you experience any of the following: stomach discomfort or soreness, clay-colored diarrhea, dark urine, lack of appetite, high temperature, cephalalgia, persistent itching, sickness and vomiting, rash, swollen legs or feet, unusual weariness, and yellow eyes or skin.

Anaphylaxis, a severe allergic reaction that can be deadly if it is not treated swiftly, can be triggered by this medicine on a very infrequent but dangerous occasion. If you or your kid has hoarseness, trouble breathing, difficulty swallowing, rash, itching, hives, or any swelling of the hands, face, or lips while taking this medicine, you should contact your doctor as soon as possible.

It has been reported that this medicine has caused serious skin reactions in certain people. Call your physician as quickly as possible if you have any changes to the skin while taking this drug, including a rash, itching, or any other changes.

If you see any changes in the regularity of your heartbeat, you should make an appointment with a physician as soon as possible. It's possible that you'll feel dizzy or faint, or that your heartbeat could become erratic, beating, or quick. It is imperative that you raise the possibility of QT prolongation or other heart rhythm problems with your primary care physician if you or a member of your family has a history of the condition.

It is conceivable that taking this drug might result in problems involving the adrenal glands. If you have symptoms such as darkening of the skin, dizziness, fainting, lack of appetite, depression, and nausea, as well as a rash, unusual lethargy or weakness, or vomiting, you should consult your doctor as soon as possible.

When using this drug, some individuals may suffer sleepiness that is not usual, dizziness, or a reduction in their level of awareness. Avoid driving large machinery until you determine how this drug works in your organism. Until then, you should not do any of those things.

Always be sure you are taking the exact dosage prescribed by your physician. Included in this are also any prescribed or OTC pharmaceuticals, including vitamins and herbs.

When deciding whether or not to use a medication responsibly, one must consider both the rewards and the risks associated with doing so. Your physician is the only one who will decide. The following considerations are important and must be kept in mind when using this medication:

Allergies

You should tell your doctor about any previous history of severe or unexpected reactions to this drug or any other medications. Be careful to let your doctor know about any additional allergies you may have in addition to those to foods, colors, or preservatives, as well as those to animals. Before you purchase something over the counter, you should make sure you are aware of what you will be receiving.

Pediatric

There does not appear to be a need for any additional safety precautions or monitoring when administering pediatric fluconazole to children ranging in age from 6 months to 13 years. However, there is insufficient evidence on the product safety and efficacy in babies younger than six months of age.

Geriatric

In the prior research that was done, fluconazole did not demonstrate any geriatric-specific concerns that might potentially limit its efficacy. Fluconazole dosage may need to be adjusted for the older population, however, because of the higher prevalence of renal problems that are associated with advancing age in this demographic.

Breastfeeding

Because there has not been an adequate amount of research done on the impact that this therapy has on human newborns, breastfeeding women should not make the assumption that there is no danger to their children from this medication. When deciding whether or not to take any medication while breastfeeding, it is critical to weigh the potential benefits against any potential risks.

Prior to take fluconazole

If you have an allergy to fluconazole, any other antifungal drugs such as itraconazole (Sporanox), ketoconazole (Nizoral), posaconazole (Noxafil), or voriconazole (Vfend), or similar or any of the components in fluconazole, you should immediately inform your physician. Check the list of products contained in the medicine.

Inform your physician if you are taking any medications that are not readily accessible in the United States, such as terfenadine (Seldane), quinidine (Quinidex), astemizole (Hismanal), cisapride (Propulsid), pimozide (Orap), quinidine (Quinidex), or erythromycin (E.E.S., E-Mycin, Erythrocin) (not for sale in the USA). If you are already on any of these medications, your physician will almost certainly urge you not to use fluconazole.

Your doctor and your pharmacist must both be informed about any other medications, such as vitamins or similar that you are now using or plan to use. In addition, you need to let your doctor know before beginning any new prescription medication if you have taken fluconazole within the last week. Include something from the following options: Calcium channel blockers (like amlodipine), warfarin (Coumadin), nifedipine, isradipine and felodipine, (Adalat, Afeditab, Procardia), carbamazepine (Carbatrol (Retrovir, in Combivir, in Trizivir). It's possible that your doctor will need to alter the amount of your medications or keep a careful check on you in case any side effects occur. Fluconazole may also interact with a large number of other medications; thus, it is imperative that you inform your physician of all the medications you are currently taking, including any that are not listed above.

Notify your doctor if you currently have or have ever had cancer, AIDS, a heartbeat that is irregular, low blood levels of calcium, salt, magnesium, or potassium, a rare genetic disorder in which the body cannot accept lactose or sucrose, heart, kidney, or liver illness, or any of these other conditions.

Informing your doctor that you are expecting is especially important during the first trimester of your pregnancy, if you are breastfeeding an infant, or if you plan to get pregnant in the near future. It is possible that your physician will recommend that you use a birth control method to avoid becoming pregnant while you are undergoing treatment and for one week after the completion of treatment. There is a chance that fluconazole will harm the fetus.

If you are about to have any kind of surgery, including dental surgery, you need to make sure that your doctor or dentist knows that you are taking fluconazole.

Fluconazole may cause seizure activity or make you feel lightheaded, so be sure you are informed of this potential side effect.

The Proper Dosage

When using this medication, be sure that you follow your physician's directions to the letter. Do not raise your dosage, increase its frequency or prolong the duration of your therapy without first consulting your doctor. All of these changes might affect the effectiveness of your treatment. If you do it, there is a greater chance that you will have some unpleasant side effects.

Take your time to read the leaflet that provides information for the patient, and be sure you follow the directions. Visit a physician if you have any worries about your health. Even if your condition starts to feel better after the first few doses of this drug, it is still very vital for you to keep taking it for the whole course of therapy. If you stop taking the antibiotic before the infection has fully cleaned up, there is a chance that it will come back. This medication may be used either with or in the absence of food.

Before putting the oral liquid to use, give it a thorough shake. For precise dosing of the drug, a spoon, an oral syringe, or a medicine cup with markings are all acceptable options. There is a possibility that a standard teaspoon will not contain the necessary liquid amount.

Different amounts of this drug are going to be necessary for different persons. Do not change for any reason the directions of your doctor.

The appropriate quantity of the medicine to take depends on its potency. The length of time that therapy is required, the number of dosages that are administered on a daily basis and the amount of time that passes in between doses are all factors that differ from one medical condition to the next.

Suspensions and pills taken by mouth:

For the initial day of therapy for cryptococcal meningitis, adults should take 400 milligrams (mg), and then continue treatment with 200 milligrams once day for at least 10 to 12 weeks. Your physician is able to adjust your dosage for you if required.

The particular child's body weight must be taken into consideration when determining the correct dose for children aged 6 months to 13 years. The suggested dosage for the first day is 12 milligrams for each kilogram of body weight. Thereafter, the recommended dosage is 6 mg per kg of body weight once daily. This particular course of therapy is carried on for a minimum of ten weeks and no more than twelve.

It is recommended that a medical expert determine the appropriate use and dose for infants and children younger than six months of age.

To treat esophageal candidiasis, adults should take a dose of 0,2 grams on the first day, followed by a dose of 0,1 grams from the second day for at least 21 days. Your doctor will establish if you require a greater dosage. The same dosage is also suitable for adults suffering with oropharyngeal candidiasis

When dealing with infections in various sections of the body:

Adults should not take doses that are more than 400 milligrams on a daily basis.

The doctor will consider the child's age as well as the child's weight when determining the proper dosage for children with ages ranging from 6 months to 13 years.

In babies less than six months, it is best to consult a medical professional on the correct application and dosage.

Adults should take 400 milligrams (mg) of the medication daily in order to lower their chances of developing candidiasis following a bone marrow transplant.

When it comes to youngsters, it is up to your doctor to decide how and how much of the medication to provide.

For adults, the recommended dosage range for treating UTIs or peritonitis is 50–200 milligrams (mg) daily.

Before administering the medication to kids, you should discuss the correct dose with their doctor.

Vaginal candidiasis treatment for adults should consist of a single dose of 150 milligrams (mg).

When it comes to youngsters, it is up to your doctor to decide how and how much of the medication to provide.

Missed Dose

If you forget to take a dose of this medicine, take it as soon as you realize that you forgot it and continue with your regular schedule. Let's say that is almost time for the next dose, than skip the dosage you forgot and restart with your scheduled doses. It is not safe to take twice the amount that is suggested.

Storage

Do not leave where children may get it.
- Do not store unnecessary or old medications.
- To find out how to properly discard of unused medication, consult your doctor.
- Put the medication in a container that won't let air in and store it somewhere where children and animals can't get to it.
- The combined oral liquid should be consumed within 14 days, whether stored in the fridge or at room temperature.

Main Side Effects

A medicine could have unintended consequences in addition to the effects that it is supposed to have. Even while not all of these negative consequences are expected to manifest themselves, in the event that they do, medical intervention could be necessary.

If you suffer any of the following bad effects, see your doctor right away:

Rare
- chest constriction
- chills
- colorless stools
- cough black urine, diarrhea, trouble swallowing, lightheartedness
- feverish heartbeat
- headache
- huge, hive-like swelling on the face, eyelids, lips, tongue, neck, hands, legs, or genitalia. itching or skin rash.
- stools with a light color
- reduced appetite
- nausea
- stomach ache, persistently bad breath, odd odor unusual, weakness or fatigue, upper right stomach or abdominal discomfort
- bloody vomiting with yellow skin and eyes
- unidentified incidence

- tarry, black stools
- skin that is flaking, peeling, or becoming loose
- chest discomfort or agony
- less urine, a dry mouth, dizziness, and hoarseness
- increased thirst, erratic or sluggish heartbeat
- muscular or joint ache
- bladder control issues
- side or lower back discomfort
- mood shifts
- cramping or aching muscles
- jerks or muscular spasms in the arms and legs
- tingling or numbness in the lips, feet, or hands
- difficult or painful urinating
- light skin
- inflamed, red eyes and red skin sores that frequently have a purple center
- seizures
- white patches or blisters in the mouth or on the lips, as well as a painful throat
- momentary unconsciousness
- enlarged glands
- uncommon bruising or bleeding

Signs of an overdose

Observing, perceiving, or feeling something that is not present as a result of having suspicion, dread, or any other form of mental alteration. There are certain possible adverse effects, most of which may be managed without the intervention of a medical professional. During the course of treatment, you may have less of these adverse reactions as your body becomes accustomed to this drug. In addition, your healthcare professional may be able to provide you advice on how to avoid or reduce the severity of some of these negative effects. Talk to your healthcare provider if any of the under listed unwanted issues persist for an extended period of time, cause you discomfort, or for any doubt you might have:

Less common
- Belching, a change in flavor, or anything unusual, unpleasant, or horrible (after) indigestion, or a stomach that is upset
- Hair thinning or shedding more of it

Additionally, there is a possibility that some persons will encounter unlisted negative effects. Talk to your doctor if you encounter any other negative effects, different from those listed above.

Pharmacist Tips for Fluconazole

- If you are using fluconazole to treat a vaginal yeast infection, you should refrain from sexual activity until your infection has been entirely cleaned up before you may resume your normal routine. When a person is suffering from an active disease, it may be exceedingly unpleasant to have sexual contact with them, and it can make their symptoms, such as burning and itching, even worse.

- It is possible to begin experiencing some amount of relief within the first twenty-four hours after initiating therapy with fluconazole (Diflucan) for a vaginal yeast infection. This is feasible after taking the medication for the first time. In the event that you don't start to feel better over the following three days, you need to get in touch with a healthcare professional as soon as possible. You may need a different dose.

- Even if you start to feel better, it is important that you finish the whole course of treatment with the fluconazole that was prescribed to you by a medical practitioner. It is possible that your infection will recur if you discontinue therapy with fluconazole (Diflucan) too soon after it has begun.

- There are a number of medicines, such as warfarin, phenytoin, and erythromycin, as well as several diabetic medications, that are known to have a detrimental interaction with fluconazole. This is by no means a full list of everything that might prevent fluconazole from functioning as intended. Always be sure that your pharmacist knows about any and all medications you are presently taking, including over-the-counter medications, and similar, especially those that require a prescription.
- You can take fluconazole either with or without food, although it should be noted that some individuals experience nausea and vomiting after taking this medication. If you discover that taking your fluconazole prescription with meals helps minimize the intensity of the side effects you don't want, try doing so the next time you take it.

Chapter 4: Combination with other Medications and Alcohol

A mild CYP2C9 and CYP3A4 inhibitor, fluconazole. Patients receiving concurrent DIFLUCAN and narrow therapeutic window medicines metabolized by CYP2C9 and CYP3A4 should be closely watched for side effects related to the concurrently given medications. The following agents/classes and DIFLUCAN have been shown to interact clinically or potentially significantly; further details are provided below:

Alfentanil
According to a research, fluconazole medication given concurrently with alfentanil caused a decrease in clearance and distribution volume as well as a prolonging of the half-life of alfentanil. Fluconazole's suppression of CYP3A4 is one potential mechanism of action. Alfentanil dosage modification can be required.

Amiodarone
Fluconazole and amiodarone treatment together may cause more QT prolongation. If fluconazole and amiodarone must

be used concurrently, caution must be used, especially when using high-dose fluconazole (800 mg).

Nortriptyline and Amitriptyline

Amitriptyline and nortriptyline are more effective when used with fluconazole. Measurements of 5-Nortriptyline and/or S-amitriptyline can be made at the beginning of combined therapy and one week afterwards. If required, the amitriptyline/nortriptyline dosage should be changed.

Amphetamine B

When given together to infected normal mice and immunosuppressed mice, fluconazole and amphotericin B had the following effects: a modest additive antifungal effect against systemic Candida albicans infection; no interaction against intracranial Cryptococcus neoformans infection; and antagonistic effects against systemic Aspergillus fumigatus infection. It is still unknown whether or if the findings of these experiments have any therapeutic relevance.

Blockers of calcium channels

Nifedipine, amlodipine, isradipine, felodipine and verapamil, are some of the calcium channel antagonists and they are reabsorbed by CYP3A4. Systemic exposure of calcium channel antagonists can be enhanced by fluconazole. It is suggested that unfavorable events be regularly monitored.

Carbamazepine

Fluconazole prevents carbamazepine from being metabolized, which results in a 30% rise in serum carbamazepine levels. Toxic reactions to carbamazepine can occur. Depending on the results of concentration measurements or the impact, carbamazepine dosage modification may be required.

Celecoxib

When fluconazole (200 mg daily) and celecoxib (200 mg) were given at the same time, the Cmax of celecoxib increased by 68%, and the AUC increased by 134%. It is possible that the dosage of celecoxib will need to be reduced by one-half when fluconazole is added.

Cyclophosphamide

The blood levels of creatinine and bilirubin rise when cyclophosphamide and fluconazole are used in combination treatment. The combination may be utilized while paying more attention to the possibility of rising blood bilirubin and creatinine levels.

Cyclosporine

With or without renal impairment, fluconazole dramatically raises cyclosporine levels in individuals undergoing renal transplantation. Patients receiving fluconazole plus cyclosporine should closely monitor their blood creatinine and cyclosporine levels. Depending on the concentration of cyclosporine, this combination may be utilized by lowering the dose.

Fentanyl

There has been one recorded fatal case of a suspected fentanyl-fluconazole combination. The patient, according to the author, passed away from fentanyl toxicity. Furthermore, it was demonstrated that fluconazole considerably slowed the clearance of fentanyl in a randomized crossover research involving 12 healthy individuals. Respiratory depression might result from elevated fentanyl content.

Inhibitors of HMG-CoA Reductase

There is a greater possibility of myopathy and rhabdomyolysis when fluconazole is used at the same time as HMG-CoA reductase inhibitors that are metabolized by CYP3A4 or CYP2C9, such as fluvastatin or atorvastatin. If it is necessary to provide concurrent therapy, the patient has to have their creatinine kinase levels examined and should be monitored for signs of myopathy and rhabdomyolysis. Stopping HMG-CoA reductase inhibitor treatment is recommended if tests reveal a considerable increase in creatinine kinase or if myopathy or rhabdomyolysis are diagnosed or suspected.

Hydrochlorothiazide

Fluconazole plasma concentrations were 40% higher when several doses of hydrochlorothiazide were given to healthy volunteers who were taking fluconazole in a pharmacokinetic interaction investigation. In patients receiving concurrent diuretics, an impact of this size shouldn't need a modification in the fluconazole dosage regimen.

Ibrutinib

Because fluconazole is a mild CYP3A4 inhibitor, it has the potential to increase plasma concentrations of ibrutinib and, as a result, the risk of experiencing adverse reactions to ibrutinib. If ibrutinib and fluconazole are administered at the same time, the recommended dosage of ibrutinib should be reduced in accordance with the prescription recommendations for ibrutinib, and the patient should be closely monitored for any adverse effects that may be caused by ibrutinib.

Lemborexant

Lemborexant's Cmax and AUC were elevated by around 1.6 and 4.2 times, respectively, when fluconazole was also administered, which is likely to enhance the likelihood of side effects such somnolence. Lemborexant should not be used concurrently with fluconazole.

Losartan

The majority of the angiotensin IL-receptor antagonism that takes place when using losartan is brought on by the active metabolite known as E-31 74, which may be stopped by taking fluconazole.

Methadone

Methadone serum levels may be increased by fluconazole. Methadone dosage change may be required.

Non-Steroidal Anti-Inflammatory Drugs

When compared to flurbiprofen administration by itself, therapy with fluconazole led to a maximum concentration (Cmax) and area under the curve (AUC) that were 23 and 81 percent higher, respectively.

Olaparib

Plasma concentrations of olaparib are raised when combined with even weak CYP3A4 inhibitors like fluconazole; hence, concurrent use is not recommended. If it is impossible to prevent the combination, your doctor may instruct you to take a lower dose of olaparib than what is recommended in the LYNPARZA (Olaparib) Prescribing Information.

Oral Contraceptives

Fluconazole has been used in two pharmacokinetic trials using an oral contraceptive that contains several doses. The 50 mg fluconazole research found no significant impact on hormone levels, but at 200 mg per day, ethinyl estradiol and levonorgestrel AUCs rose by 40% and 24%, respectively.

Oral Hypoglycemics

The combination of fluconazole with oral hypoglycemic medications has been linked to one fatality from hypoglycemia; clinically severe hypoglycemia may be triggered by both medications. Fluconazole raises the plasma levels of tolbutamide, glyburide, and glipizide while decreasing their metabolism. Blood glucose levels should be closely watched when fluconazole is administered concurrently with these or other sulfonylurea oral hypoglycemic medications, and the sulfonylurea dose should be changed as appropriate.

Phenytoin

Phenytoin plasma concentrations are raised with fluconazole. It is advised that patients receiving fluconazole with phenytoin have their phenytoin levels carefully monitored.

Pimozide

Fluconazole with pimozide dosing together has not been tested *in vitro or in vivo,* however it may impede pimozide metabolism. Infrequent incidences of *torsade de pointes* and QT prolongation can result from elevated pimozide plasma concentrations. Fluconazole and pimozide should not be administered together.

Prednisone

According to a case study, a patient who had a liver transplant and was on prednisone who stopped taking fluconazole after three months experienced severe adrenal cortical insufficiency. Fluconazole withdrawal is thought to have boosted CYP3A4 activity, which increased prednisone metabolism. When fluconazole is stopped, patients who are receiving prednisone plus fluconazole for a prolonged period of time should have their adrenal cortical insufficiency closely checked.

Quinidine

Fluconazole with quinidine given together has not been tested *in vitro or in vivo*, however it may decrease quinidine metabolism. There have been isolated cases of *torsade de pointes* and QT prolongation linked to quinidine use. Quinidine and fluconazole should not be administered together.

Rifabutin

According to some accounts, there is an interaction when fluconazole and rifabutin are given at the same time that results in up to 80% higher rifabutin blood levels. Uveitis has been reported in individuals who had fluconazole and rifabutin at the same time. Patients getting rifabutin and fluconazole at the same time need to be closely watched.

Rifampin

Rifampin speeds up the metabolism of fluconazole when it is taken at the same time. Consideration should be made to raising the dose of fluconazole when it is delivered together with rifampin, depending on the clinical situation.

Saquinavir

Fluconazole inhibits P-glycoprotein and reduces the clearance of saquinavir by about 50%. This is because fluconazole suppresses the hepatic metabolism of saquinavir via CYP3A4 and increases the AUC and Cmax of saquinavir. Saquinavir clearance is reduced because fluconazole increases its AUC and Cmax. Saquinavir dose modification can be necessary.

Benzodiazepines with a Short Acting

After buccal administration of midazolam, fluconazole produced a considerable rise in both the concentrations of the drug and its psychomotor issues. It would indicate that taking fluconazole orally has a higher influence on the effects of midazolam than receiving the medication intravenously. If a combination of fluconazole and short-acting benzodiazepines, both of which are metabolized by the cytochrome P450 system, is administered to a patient, the dosage of the short-acting benzodiazepines should be decreased, and the patient should be monitored very closely.

Sirolimus

Fluconazole raises sirolimus plasma concentrations likely through preventing sirolimus from being metabolized by CYP3A4 and P-glycoprotein. Depending on the effect/concentration readings, sirolimus dose may need to be adjusted while using this combo.

Tacrolimus

Due to the suppression of tacrolimus metabolism by CYP3A4 in the intestines caused by fluconazole, the blood concentrations of tacrolimus taken orally may increase by up to 5 times. When tacrolimus is administered intravenously, no notable pharmacokinetic alterations have been noticed. Tacrolimus levels, that are higher, have been linked to nephrotoxicity.The dosage of tacrolimus must be adjusted according to its concentration.

Theophylline

Theophylline serum concentrations are raised with fluconazole. In patients using fluconazole with theophylline, careful monitoring of serum theophylline concentrations is advised.

Tofacitinib

When tofacitinib and fluconazole are delivered together, tofacitinib systemic exposure is enhanced. When taken together with fluconazole, tofacitinib dosage should be decreased.

Tolvaptan

Plasma exposure to tolvaptan is considerably increased when fluconazole, a weak CYP3A4 inhibitor, is supplied simultaneously with tolvaptan, a CYP3A4 substrate. This results in a higher concentration of tolvaptan in the plasma. Because of the interaction between these two drugs, there is a potentially considerable increase in the risk of adverse effects associated with tolvaptan, including major diuresis, dehydration, and acute renal failure.

Vinca Alkaloids

Although fluconazole has not been thoroughly researched, it may cause neurotoxicity through increasing plasma levels of vinca alkaloids (such as vincristine and vinblastine).

Voriconazole

Do not provide fluconazole and voriconazole together. Voriconazole toxicity and adverse event monitoring are advised, particularly if voriconazole is begun less than 24 hours following the previous dosage of fluconazole.

Interaction with Alcohol

Fluconazole and alcohol do not interact, however it is typically not advised to consume alcohol while recuperating from an infection. Alcohol has a tendency to impair immunological response, at least temporarily. Additionally, it may exacerbate negative drug side effects like:

- Nausea.
- Diarrhea.
- uneasy stomach

Fluconazole stays in the body for six to ten days, which is a long time. You would need to wait that amount of time if you wanted to fully avoid drinking while the medication is present.

Does Alcohol Consumption Reduce the Effectiveness of fluconazole?

Does the use of alcohol render the antifungal medication fluconazole useless, despite the fact that it is not suggested that you combine the two substances due to the increased risk of liver damage and intensified symptoms?

The widespread misconception that drinking alcohol makes antibiotics useless has caused a significant number of individuals to inquire about this topic. This is not accurate, and consuming alcohol while taking fluconazole does not render the medication ineffective in any way. It is possible that it will result in undesirable side effects, but one of those effects will not be ineffectiveness.

People may also question if alcohol might return fluconazole ineffective because of the impact that it has on the immune system. This is another reason why people may ask if alcohol can have this effect. Since alcohol consumption has the effect of suppressing the immune system, drinking might make it more difficult for you to recover from the infection that brought you to require the use of fluconazole in the first place. It's possible that this will lead you to believe that drinking alcohol will render fluconazole ineffective, but in truth, the medication is just as effective as it would be under normal circumstances.

When considering the interaction between alcohol and fluconazole, it is essential to keep in mind not only the possibility of increased adverse effects and toxicity to the liver, but also the requirement that your body be healthy in order to repair itself.

Chapter 5: Pregnancy and Breastfeeding

Is it possible and safe to use Fluconazole when pregnant?

Using Fluconazole while Pregnant

Animal studies using high doses have shown signs of teratogenicity, fetotoxicity, and embryolethality.

Numerous epidemiological studies indicate that there is no correlation between low-dose exposure during pregnancy and an increased incidence of congenital malformations. The majority of patients got a single oral dosage of 150 milligrams, and these individuals were the focus of these investigations. There was no evidence of any adverse effects on the developing baby in the data collected from several hundred pregnant women who took standard doses (less than 200 mg per day) either once or several times throughout the first trimester of their pregnancies.

During her pregnancy, a woman who was treated for disseminated coccidioidomycosis with a daily dose of 400 mg gave birth to a daughter who was born prematurely and had abnormalities. The infant was born with several physical abnormalities, including a cleft palate, a bowed tibia and femur, humeral-radial fusion, bilateral femoral fractures, contractures of the upper and lower limbs, and digit deformities. A congenital abnormality was the root of each of these illnesses from the beginning. Complications from frontal bone cranioschisis, sagittal suture craniostenosis, to nasal bone hypoplasia, caused the infant's untimely death shortly after birth.

It was discovered that there were two additional instances of congenital malformations in infants who were born to women who used this medicine at any point during or after the first trimester of their pregnancies. There were anomalies found in the skeleton, the heart, and the craniofacial region. There was just one infant who survived. A Candida albicans sepsis was successfully treated in a pregnant woman who was 24 years old and in the 16th week of her pregnancy by giving her this medicine. She received a total of 10 mg/kg over the course of 50 days. The patient's sepsis was successfully treated, and the remainder of the pregnancy proceeded properly. At the 39th week of her pregnancy, she gave birth to a girl who was perfectly healthy and shown no signs of any congenital problems. At the age of two, the child's physical growth and brain development were completely normal.

A group of 170,453 pregnant women who did not fill any prescriptions for fluconazole during their pregnancies was compared to a group of 1079 pregnant women who gave birth alive or had a stillbirth after the 20th week of gestation and who had filled at least one prescription for this medication. The ladies were chosen based on their entries in the Danish Medical Birth Registry. The information on drug use, birth outcomes, and confounders was gathered from databases that were population-based and focused on healthcare. 797 (74%) of the 1079 women who took this medicine during the first trimester were given 150 milligrams, 235 (22%) were given 300 milligrams, 24 (2%), 350 milligrams, and 23 (2%), 600 milligrams. The other women were given either 350 milligrams or 600 milligrams. The babies born to these mothers had a total of 44 (4.1%) cases of congenital abnormalities. Congenital abnormalities were present in 6,152 (3.6%) of the 170,453 babies who were delivered to moms who did not have prescriptions for fluconazole. According to the findings of the study, using this medicine for a limited amount of time during the first trimester of pregnancy did not appear to increase the overall risk of congenital defects in the offspring.

Medications that have been shown to increase the risk of fetal abnormalities or irreversible injury, or those are suspected of doing so, fall under the AU TGA's pregnancy category D classification. There is a possibility that these medicines will have unfavorable pharmacological effects. Please refer to the supplementary materials for any further information you may want.

Even though there are not enough well-controlled human trials, and animal reproduction studies have shown that the medicine has a deleterious effect on the developing baby, it is possible that the benefits of using the medication during pregnancy exceed the potential dangers to the unborn child.

According to the US Food and Drug Administration's (FDA) pregnancy category D, which states that there is positive evidence of a human fetal risk based on data on adverse reactions from investigational, marketing experience or human studies, the drug may still be used during pregnancy due to the possibility of benefits despite the possibility of risks.

Use should be avoided until there is sufficient evidence that the benefits outweigh the risks to the developing fetus, with the exception of severe or potentially deadly fungal infections.

- In the United Kingdom, conventional doses and short-term therapy are not recommended, unless the patient has an illness that might potentially be deadly. High-dose and/or prolonged treatment regimens should not be utilized during pregnancy.
- Pregnancy category under AU TGA: D

Using Fluconazole while Breastfeeding

The amounts of this medicine that are excreted in human milk are either lower than those seen in maternal plasma or are on par with those levels. Breast milk contains far less of the drug than is given to newborns.

Breast candidiasis is a common condition that affects nursing mothers, and this medicine is commonly prescribed to treat it. The Academy of Breastfeeding Medicine notes that this prescription is particularly useful in cases when the infection is persistent or recurring. However, fluconazole has not been subjected to sufficient research in the treatment of Candida mastitis. It is common practice to give this drug to the mother and the infant at the same time in the event that other therapies are unsuccessful. In most cases, an initial dose of 400 milligrams is administered, and then the patient is instructed to take 200 milligrams daily for at least two weeks or until the pain subsides; however, in one study conducted in Australia, the participants were given 150 milligrams every other day until the breast discomfort subsided. The quantity of fluconazole that is produced in breast milk by the mother at these doses is insufficient to cure oral thrush in the nursing newborn.

On day 20 following delivery, the peak milk level in a woman who took 200 milligrams orally once a day for 18 days was of 4.1 milligrams per liter two hours after the dose; the average-life of excretion from breast milk was 26.9 hours. The day 20 after the lady had given birth was when the milk production reached its highest level. Another mother took a single oral dose of 150 mg twelve weeks after giving birth to one of her children. The greatest quantities of the drug in the milk were found two and five hours after the injection, with corresponding readings of 2.9 and 2.7 milligrams per liter. The levels of the medication in the milk were 1.8 milligrams per liter 24 hours after the treatment, and 1 milligram per liter 48 hours after the dose. Milk contained roughly a medication with an average life of more or less 30 hours. This is sixty percent of the recommended dose for neonates younger than two weeks old and twenty percent of the dose used in older infants for the treatment of oral thrush.

This was the case in a woman who received a single oral dose of 150 mg to treat vaginal candidiasis. A dosage of 150 milligrams taken orally was administered to the lady in order to treat vaginal candidiasis.

The women who participated in the clinical study of this drug for the treatment of thrush of the breasts that is connected with nursing were instructed to take an average of 7.3 capsules of 150 mg daily until the discomfort subsided. 7 women of the group reported adverse effects in their infants that may possibly be attributable to fluconazole. These problems included diarrhea, vomiting, and stomach pain. These adverse effects included flushing of the cheeks, discomfort in the gastrointestinal tract, and diarrhea or diarrhea with mucus.

At least two infants received a dose of 6 mg/kg. There was a little and momentary rise in the infant's liver function tests, but this increase went down once the infant's dosage was lowered. The increase in the infant's liver function tests was negligible. These instances demonstrate that this drug may be properly supplied while breastfeeding because newborns would receive a far lower amount of the medication; nevertheless, further experience is still required to determine whether or not it is safe.

Consequences of using Fluconazole when pregnant or breastfeeding

It is perfectly safe for nursing mothers to take the antifungal medicine fluconazole since the quantity of the drug that is excreted into breast milk is a far lower amount than the dose that is given to infants. It is common practice to prescribe the medication fluconazole to nursing mothers who suffer from breast candidiasis. This is done despite the fact that there have been no good clinical studies reported on fluconazole effectiveness in treating Candida mastitis. Clinical trials on fluconazole effectiveness in treating Candida mastitis have not been reported. This is mainly found whenever the infection continues to exist or returns often. When various forms of treatment have been explored and proven failed, it is common practice to try treating both the mother and the kid with fluconazole. When given to mothers, the normal dosage is 400 milligrams all at once, followed by 200 mg daily for at least two weeks or until the disease is gone. On the other hand, one research project that was carried out in Australia utilized a dosage of 150 milligrams every other day till the breast discomfort was over. Oral thrush in neonates cannot be effectively treated by breast-feeding at the present maternal concentrations because there are insufficient amounts of fluconazole that are detected in breast milk.

In a trial that investigated the efficacy of fluconazole in treating thrush of the breasts brought on by nursing, the researchers had the moms take an average of 7.3 capsules (range: 1-29) of 150 mg every other day until the discomfort was gone. Seven of the 96 women who nursed their children reported unfavorable effects in those youngsters that may have been caused by the fluconazole they were taking. In addition to rashes, these symptoms included nausea, vomiting, and diarrhea. A flushing of the cheeks, pain in the stomach, and bowel motions that were either loose or bloody were some of the symptoms.

Chapter 6: Frequently Asked Questions

1) What infections does Fluconazole treat?

Fluconazole is a medication that is prescribed for the treatment of acute yeast infections (fungal infections), such as vaginal candidiasis, pharyngo-oral and esophageal candidiasis, and other similar disorders, such as urinary system infections, peritonitis, and infections that may affect different parts of the body. Patients who are having bone marrow transplants, as well as those who are undergoing radiation treatment or chemotherapy, have the option of using fluconazole to prevent candidiasis.

2) Which is the perfect way to take Fluconazole?

Fluconazole comes in tablet and liquid form, both of which can be consumed at any point throughout the day, regardless of food intake. There are three main dosage levels of fluconazole that are available in capsule form: 50 milligrams (mg), 150 milligrams (mg), and 200 milligrams (mg). After taking the tablets in the prescribed manner, wash them down with a full glass of water. Always remember to take your medication at the same time each day for the best possible outcomes.

3) Is Fluconazole an antibiotic?

Fluconazole is an antifungal specifically used to treat either systemic and superficial fungal infections in many bodily systems.

4) Is Fluconazole safe to take during the three last months of pregnancy?

Since the risk of miscarriage has passed by 20 weeks and the baby's heart is completely established by 12 weeks, using fluconazole in the third trimester would not be able to create difficulties. There is no evidence that using fluconazole during pregnancy increases the risk of stillbirth, premature delivery, or low birth weight.

5) Can Fluconazole be used to treat ringworm?

Oral fluconazole medication appears to be safe, according to studies. The results of this trial showed that a 150-mg weekly dosage of oral fluconazole was successful in treating cutaneous candidosis, *tinea corporis, tinea cruris, and tinea pedis.*

6) Is there a specific time to use Fluconazole?

It doesn't matter if you take fluconazole before or after a meal, because it works the same either way. For certain diseases, such vaginal thrush, a single 150 mg dosage is sufficient to clear the illness, while others may require many weeks of therapy.

7) What are the side effects of Fluconazole?

Hair loss, nausea, vomiting, diarrhea, stomach discomfort or pain, headache, and dizziness are all possible side effects. Notify your healthcare provider or pharmacist immediately if these symptoms are persisting or even getting worse.

Remind that your doctor prescribed this drug after a careful examination of risks and benefit of using it.

Extreme adverse effects, such as a rapid or irregular heartbeat, severe dizziness, or fainting, require immediate medical attention.

Rarely, but possibly, this medicine may induce severe liver damage. A person who has persistent nausea and vomiting, severe stomach or abdominal pain, yellowing of the eyes or skin, or black urine should seek medical attention immediately.

Exceptionally acute allergic reactions to this drug are rare. If persistent fever, new or worsening lymph node enlargement, rash, itching, swelling of tongue or throat, dizziness, or difficulty breathing occur, call your doctor immediately.

8) How often can you take Fluconazole?

It is recommended that you take fluconazole once a day. The severity of your infection will determine both the strength of your medication and how long you will need to take it. Taking fluconazole with or without meals is OK.

9) After a therapy with Fluconazole, how long do you have to wait before drinking alcohol?

Considering that it can induce acute stomach disease such as cramps, nausea and vomiting, you should avoid consuming alcoholic drinks while taking this drug and for at least 3 days after you cease using it.

10) If symptoms persist after using Fluconazole, what else can be done?

If, after taking fluconazole for a week, your symptoms have not improved, you should make an appointment with your primary care physician.

11) How effective is Fluconazole against fungal skin infections?

Even at lesser dosages, fluconazole is particularly efficient at reducing superficial fungal infections. Despite an increase in colonization, there has been no rise in the confirmed, systemic infection of fungi that are resistant to fluconazole.

12) How fast does Fluconazole work?

Depending on what purpose you're using it for. You might only take one dosage of fluconazole to treat a vaginal yeast infection, and you could start to feel better within 24 hours. For further instructions, speak with your healthcare physician if your symptoms don't go away in 3 days. Another dosage could be necessary.

Before you start to feel better, it might take several days for certain other illnesses (such oral thrush). It could take longer for infections that are more severe, such those that affect the blood or liver.

You should continue taking fluconazole until your prescription is fulfilled, even if you start to feel better. An early interruption of the drug may not lead to the complete recovery.

This can make the infection symptoms come back.

13) Is Fluconazole water soluble?

Protein binding for fluconazole is quite low. Fluconazole, unlike certain other azoles, is more water-soluble, meaning it may move through bodily fluids including saliva, urine, synovial fluid, and cerebrospinal fluid (CSF).

14) Can I use cannabis while taking Fluconazole?

Patients using fluconazole are cautioned not to use cannabis. The risk of harmful effects from some cannabinoids may rise if they are exposed to other cannabinoids at the same time.

15) How long can you take Fluconazole?

Whether you should stop or not taking fluconazole depends on what caused your illness and how well it is responding to the treatment. It may consist of a single dose or a course of therapy that would run for a few weeks, months, or even years. If your physician prescribes fluconazole for you, they will also specify the length of time you have to take the medication. You should keep taking your prescription until the prescribed amount of time has passed, even if you start to feel better. This will prevent future relapsing of the disease. In order to treat infections, fluconazole is often administered for just a limited amount of time. If you have a serious disease, your doctor may recommend that you continue taking fluconazole for a very long period. It is safe for you to continue taking it for an extended period of time if your physician has advised you to do so. Before you discontinue taking any medicine for whatever reason, you should discuss your decision with your primary care physician.